ESSENTIAL CHRONIC LYMPHOCYTIC LEUKEMIA DIET

The CLL Cookbook: Dietary Solutions For Patients With CLL, Fostering Revitalization, Nourishment, And Restoration

NEIL CASSIUS

1

Table of Contents

Introductory

Cancer of the blood and bone marrow, known as chronic lymphocytic leukemia (CLL). Lymphocytes, which are part of the body's immune system, proliferate and accumulate abnormally in excessive numbers, marking this condition. Because of this, CLL tends to worsen gradually over time.

White blood cells called lymphocytes play an important role in the body's defense against pathogens. Bone marrow, lymph nodes, and other organs fill up with CLL's dysfunctional lymphocytes. Anemia, increased susceptibility to infections, and excessive bleeding can result from a surplus of these aberrant cells, which interfere with the synthesis of healthy blood cells including red blood cells and platelets.

Although the precise reason why certain people are more likely to develop CLL than others is still unknown, we know that genetic variations and family history are among them. The average age of diagnosis is roughly 70, making it a disease primarily of the elderly.

CLL symptoms can be vague or nonexistent at first, depending on the patient. Common signs and symptoms include weakness, swollen lymph nodes, night sweats, a loss of appetite, recurrent infections, and a propensity to bruise or bleed easily. However, CLL is typically found via routine blood testing because some people with the disease may go without symptoms for a long time.

A bone marrow biopsy is used to confirm the presence of abnormal lymphocytes after a physical examination and blood tests have indicated the existence of CLL. The progression of the disease, measured by the number of accumulated lymphocytes and other criteria, informs the choice of treatment.

The severity of symptoms, the extent of the disease, and the patient's general health all play a role in determining the best course of treatment for chronic lymphocytic leukemia (CLL).

A "watch and wait" strategy, where the disease is monitored on a regular basis but not treated right away, may be implemented in the early stages when there are no or few symptoms. Chemotherapy, targeted therapy, immunotherapy, and stem cell transplantation are all potential treatment options.

The prognosis for chronic lymphocytic leukemia (CLL) varies

according to a number of factors, including the patient's age, general health, disease progression, and response to treatment. While some people with CLL may have a mild disease history and go years without therapy, others may have a more aggressive type of the disease that needs to be monitored constantly.

In order to track the course of the condition and make any necessary adjustments to the treatment plan, regular checkups with a healthcare expert are essential.

CHAPTER ONE
Factors And Causes

Chronic lymphocytic leukemia (CLL) has mysterious underpinnings. On the other hand, various risk factors and contributors to the development of CLL have been discovered. Among these are the following:

• Increased risk of CLL has been linked to specific genetic variants. TP53, ATM, NOTCH1, and SF3B1 gene mutations are frequently observed in CLL patients. These changes can cause cellular dysfunction, which is a key factor in the progression of leukemia.

• Having a parent or sibling who was diagnosed with CLL or another lymphoid cancer raises your risk for having the disease. This elevated risk may result from a combination of hereditary susceptibility and environmental factors that tend to run in families.

• Age: CLL strikes the elderly more often than younger people. The typical age of diagnosis is roughly 70 years old, and the likelihood of having CLL rises with age. CLL is extremely uncommon in people under the age of 40.

• The incidence of CLL is somewhat higher in males than in females. It is unclear what causes this disparity between the sexes.

• A higher risk of developing CLL has been linked to exposure to a number of pollutants, including benzene and certain herbicides and pesticides. However, further research is needed to determine the precise connection between these substances and CLL.

• Immune System Dysfunction: People with HIV/AIDS or autoimmune illnesses may be at a higher risk of getting CLL than the general population. This points to immune system dysfunction as a potential cause of the disease.

Although these variables may raise the likelihood of having CLL, many people who are diagnosed with the disease have no known risk factors. The exact role of genetic, environmental, and other variables in the progression of CLL is still being investigated, and the disease can arise in people for whom no risk factors are recognized.

Strategies For Treatment

Factors such as the severity of symptoms, the patient's general health, and the genetic or molecular characteristics of the CLL cells all play a role in determining the best course of treatment.

The treatment's aims may include disease management, symptom alleviation, quality of life enhancement, and even survival extension. Common methods of dealing with CLL include:

• A "watch and wait" strategy may be taken in the early stages of CLL, when no or few symptoms are present. Regular checkups and blood tests are performed to keep an eye on the condition without starting treatment right away. When the disease advances or noticeable symptoms appear, treatment can begin.

• Chemotherapy is the practice of using medications to inhibit the growth of cancer cells. Fludarabine, cyclophosphamide, and bendamustine are examples of standard chemotherapy medicines that can be administered singly or in combination.

Both oral and intravenous forms of chemotherapy are available, and both are often provided in cycles, with breaks between treatments to allow the body to heal.

• Targeted therapy refers to the use of medications to inhibit the development and survival of CLL cells by focusing on specific molecules or processes.

Monoclonal antibodies like rituximab, obinutuzumab, and ofatumumab are examples of targeted therapy utilized in CLL. These antibodies can either directly suppress the proliferation of CLL cells by binding to certain proteins on their surface or flag them for elimination by the immune system.

• Immunotherapy is a treatment method that encourages the immune system to identify and eliminate cancer cells. Immune checkpoint inhibitors, such as pembrolizumab and nivolumab, are used as part of immunotherapy for CLL. These drugs help to release the brakes on the immune system, allowing it to more effectively attack cancer cells.

• Ibrutinib and acalabrutinib are examples of Bruton's tyrosine kinase (BTK) inhibitors, which are oral targeted medicines that reduce the activity of the BTK enzyme. In patients with specific genetic alterations, these medications have demonstrated to be highly beneficial in the treatment of CLL.

- Stem cell transplantation (also known as bone marrow transplantation) may be an option for individuals with aggressive or recurrent CLL who are young and otherwise healthy. A donor's healthy stem cells are inserted into the patient's damaged bone marrow to stimulate the creation of new, healthy blood cells.

- Clinical TrialsEnrolling in a clinical trial is one way to gain access to experimental treatments for CLL. Patients who have not responded to normal therapies may have more options thanks to the findings of clinical studies, which assist increase medical knowledge.

Many variables influence the therapy path taken, and each patient's care is tailored to their unique disease presentation and health status.

Research and development of innovative medicines, including as combination methods and customized therapy based on genetic profiling, are constantly altering the terrain of CLL treatment. Patients need to have open communication with their healthcare providers about their concerns and desired outcomes during therapy.

CHAPTER TWO
Diet's Impact On Controlling CLL

Although nutrition is an important factor in the management of Chronic Lymphocytic Leukemia (CLL), it is vital to keep in mind that diet alone cannot cure or directly treat CLL.

However, keeping up a nutritious diet can help the body function, the immune system, and the well-being of the patient as a whole while undergoing CLL therapy. The following are some dietary suggestions that may help:

• Eat a wide range of fruits, vegetables, whole grains, lean meats, and healthy fats to achieve a healthy, balanced diet. This has the potential to supply vitamins, minerals, and other nutrients that are crucial to good health. Eat a rainbow of fruits and vegetables to absorb a wide spectrum of antioxidants and lower your chance of developing certain malignancies.

• Staying well-hydrated is essential, so make sure you drink plenty of water and other fluids. Water is essential to the body and plays a role in keeping it healthy and functioning properly. Constipation and nausea are two medication side effects that can be mitigated by drinking enough water.

• Whole grains, legumes, fruits, and vegetables are all great examples of high-fiber foods that should be incorporated into your daily diet. Certain therapies can cause constipation, which fiber can help alleviate or at least manage.

• Select healthy fats from foods like avocados, nuts, seeds, and olive oil. These fats are a good source of heart-healthy essential fatty acids.

• Foods High in Protein Be sure to eat a variety of lean protein foods such fish, poultry, beans, and tofu. During cancer treatment, protein is essential for tissue repair and maintenance.

• Consume less processed meals because of their high levels of harmful fats, sodium, and added sugars. These meals are not good for you and may even cause you to gain weight or have other health problems.

• Customized Treatment Plan: Consult with an oncology-trained registered dietician. They can tailor their advice to your condition, treatment plan, and any obstacles you face in the kitchen.

Dietary changes alone are not a replacement for medical care, however. Dietary recommendations may be part of your healthcare team's advise and recommendations for managing CLL. The advice they give you will be tailored to your individual health status and treatment plan.

Formulating A Food Plan To Fight Cll

When planning a diet to help with CLL, it is most crucial to include foods that are high in nutrients and good for your health in general. The following suggestions can help you make healthy food choices even though there are no CLL-specific dietary guidelines:

• Eat at least five servings of fruits and vegetables every day, preferably a wide variety. Vitamins, minerals, and antioxidants abound in these foods, making them beneficial to your immune system and general well-being. Choose a rainbow of produce for a wide range of vitamins and minerals.

• Brown rice, quinoa, whole wheat bread, and oats are all examples of whole grains that you should include in your diet. Vitamins, minerals, and dietary fiber are all provided. Whole grains can help with both digestion and keeping your energy levels consistent.

• Include lean protein sources like chicken, fish, beans, tofu, and Greek yogurt in your diet. Protein is required for normal cellular growth, cell division, and immune system function. Protein sources like fish, which are rich in omega-3 fatty acids, which may have anti-inflammatory effects, should be included if they are compatible with your treatment plan or personal preferences.

• Avocados, almonds, seeds, and olive oil are all examples of healthy fats that you should incorporate into your diet. These fats are a good source of heart-healthy essential fatty acids. However, keep in mind that fats are high in calories, so moderation is key.

• Drink plenty of water throughout the day to keep yourself hydrated. Maintaining a healthy fluid balance is important for general well-being and can reduce the severity of treatment-related side effects including nausea and constipation.

• Avoid eating too many processed foods because they are typically high in harmful fats, salt, and added sugars. Instead, eat more complete, unprocessed foods to get the most out of your diet.

• Treatment and management of CLL can be different for each individual patient. You might want to talk to a dietician who focuses on cancer patients. They can tailor their advice to your condition, treatment plan, and dietary limitations or difficulties.

• Think About Supplements: Before beginning any supplement regimen, it is essential to discuss it with your healthcare providers.

While eating a healthy, well-rounded diet should meet most people's nutritional requirements, supplements may be necessary for those with special dietary requirements. If you have questions about whether or not you should take supplements, talk to your healthcare team.

Keep in mind that your healthcare team is in the best position to advise you on your diet depending on your individual condition and treatment plan. To provide the best possible care, they will take into account any interactions between your diet, drugs, and treatment plans.

CHAPTER THREE
Included Foods

Include foods that are high in nutrients and beneficial to your health and well-being as part of a CLL-friendly diet. Some examples of appropriate foods to add:

• Berries such as blueberries, strawberries, raspberries, and blackberries are high in phytochemicals and antioxidants, both of which may help prevent cancer. Additionally, they contain a lot of fiber.

• Broccoli, cauliflower, kale, cabbage, and Brussels sprouts are all examples of cruciferous vegetables. These veggies are a good source of vitamins, minerals, and fiber, and they also contain chemicals that may have anti-cancer benefits.

• Vitamin C, which is abundant in citrus fruits including oranges, grapefruits, lemons, and limes, is thought to have antioxidant characteristics and aid in immune system function. Both water and fiber can be found in them.

• Spinach, kale, Swiss chard, and arugula are just some examples of leafy greens that you should add to your diet. Vitamins, minerals, and antioxidants abound in these greens, making them beneficial for one's health as a whole. Salads, smoothies, and prepared meals can all benefit from their incorporation.

• Veggies with Lots of ColorInclude a rainbow of veggies in your diet, from bell peppers and tomatoes to carrots and sweet potatoes and beets. Vitamins, minerals, and antioxidants abound in these greens, helping to strengthen your immune system and promote general wellness.

• Brown rice, quinoa, whole wheat bread, and oats are all examples of whole grains that you should eat. They include beneficial nutrients including fiber and vitamins and minerals and can aid in controlling blood sugar and facilitating digestion.

• Skinless chicken, fish, beans, tofu, and Greek yogurt are all great lean protein options. Protein is crucial for maintaining health, repairing damaged tissues, and boosting the immune system.

• Avocados, nuts (almonds, walnuts), seeds (chia seeds, flaxseeds), and olive oil are all great examples of healthy fats that can be incorporated into your diet. These fats are a good source of heart-healthy essential fatty acids.

• Green Tea: Compounds in green tea have been investigated for their possible anticancer effects. It may be preferable to sugary drinks in some cases.

• Hydrate yourself during the day by drinking plenty of water. Keeping yourself well-hydrated is crucial to your health and can reduce the severity of any adverse effects from your therapy.

It is important to consult with your healthcare team or an oncology-trained registered dietitian to create a diet plan tailored to your needs, treatment plan, and any dietary limitations or obstacles you may face.

They can give you personalized advice and encouragement to help you pick the foods that are best for your health.

Restrictive Or Prohibited Foods

It is vital to remember to limit or avoid specific foods while creating a CLL-friendly diet. Some things to keep in mind are:

• Restrict your intake of processed foods such as packaged snacks, fizzy drinks, sweets, and even processed meats. These foods are linked to inflammation, weight gain, and other health problems due to their high quantities of harmful fats, sodium, and added sugars.

• Lessen your consumption of red and processed meats like beef, lamb, and pork as well as other options like sausage, bacon, and deli meats. There may be adverse health effects and an elevated risk of some cancers from eating these foods. Instead, try eating more lean proteins like those found in poultry, fish, lentils, and other plant foods.

• Foods high in trans fats should be avoided or consumed in moderation. Fried foods, processed snacks, and professionally baked items are typical sources of these lipids. Inflammation, cardiovascular disease, and other illnesses may all be exacerbated by trans fats.

• Consuming excessive amounts of alcohol can compromise your immune system, cause harmful drug interactions, and lead to dehydration, among other health problems. If you prefer to drink alcohol, do so moderately and discuss any concerns you may have with your healthcare provider.

• Avoid high-sodium items like processed snacks, canned soups, and fast meals to keep your salt intake in check. Too much sodium has been linked to fluid retention and hypertension.

• Choose organic versions of commonly eaten fruits and vegetables to reduce your exposure to pesticides. You can also lessen your risk of being exposed to pesticides by washing conventionally cultivated produce thoroughly.

• Personal Factors: Think about any nutritional advice your doctor or healthcare team has given you. Depending on your treatment plan, drugs, and personal circumstances, they may recommend that you avoid particular foods or dietary groups.

Since everyone is different in terms of their health, treatment plan, and dietary preferences, it is best to speak with a certified dietitian who specializes in cancer nutrition for tailored advice. They will guide you through the maze of nutritional issues to help you make the best decisions for your health.

CHAPTER FOUR
Recipes For The Morning Meal

Some breakfast options that are CLL-friendly, along with recipes, include as follows:

1. Parfait with Berries and Yogurt:

• Ingredients:

• One cup of Greek yogurt (regular or fruit-flavored).

• Strawberries, blueberries, and raspberries, oh my!

• Toasted granola with chopped nuts.

• Honey.

Instructions:

• Greek yogurt, granola, or crushed almonds can be layered in a glass or bowl with a variety of fruit.

• Continue layering until all of the ingredients are gone.

• Honey can be drizzled on top if desired.

• Have fun with the healthy and tasty parfait.

2. Eggs with Vegetables:

• **Ingredients:**

• 2 eggs.

- Veggie medley (broccoli, cauliflower, tomatoes, bell peppers, mushrooms, etc.).

- To taste, salt and pepper.

- Oil from olives or nonstick spray.

Instructions:

- Coat a nonstick pan with olive oil or cooking spray and heat it over medium heat.

- Salt and pepper the eggs after you have whisked them in a bowl.

- Cook the mixed vegetables until they are just soft in a pan.

• Fold the omelette in half and pour the eggs over the veggies to cook until the eggs are set.

• Put the omelette on a hot plate by sliding it there.

3. Recipe for Chia Seed Pudding:

• Ingredients:

• Chia seeds, about 2 tablespoons.

• 1 cup of almond milk (or your preferred milk).

• One teaspoon of honey or maple syrup.

• Sliced bananas, berries, or mango chunks for topping.

Instructions:

- Combine the chia seeds, almond milk, and sugar in a sealed container.

- Make sure the chia seeds are spread out by stirring them thoroughly.

- To make a pudding-like consistency from the chia seeds, cover the jar or bowl and place it in the fridge for at least 4 hours, preferably overnight.

- Put your favorite fruits on top of the pudding and stir it up when it is time to serve.

- Have a satisfying meal of chia pudding.

Do not forget to customize the recipe to your tastes and dietary restrictions by adjusting the serving quantities and components. You can make these recipes your own by adding or removing items to suit your personal preferences and dietary needs.

Suggestions For Lunch And Dinner

Here are some meal ideas and recipes to consider if you have CLL:

1. Salad with Grilled Chicken:

• **Ingredients:**

• Slices of grilled chicken breast.

greens for salad (spinach, romaine, arugula, etc.)

• Sliced or halved cherry tomatoes.

• Sliced Cucumber.

• Cubed Avocado.

• Nuts, seeds, and feta cheese can be used as a topping.

Dressing:

• Oil from olives.

• To Use: o Vinegar or Lemon Juice.

• To taste, salt and pepper.

Instructions:

• Chopped avocado, cherry tomatoes, cucumber, and mixed salad greens should all be combined together in a big bowl.

• Add grilled chicken slices and other toppings like seeds, almonds, and feta cheese to the salad.

• The dressing can be made in a separate small bowl by whisking all the ingredients together.

• You may either toss the salad with the dressing or serve it on the side.

• Gently toss the salad to mix all the ingredients and savor a healthy and refreshing lunch.

2. Salmon with vegetables baked in the oven:

• Ingredients:

• Filet of salmon.

• Broccoli, cauliflower, carrots, and bell peppers, among others.

• Oil from olives.

• Lemon juice.

• Powdered garlic.

• To taste, salt and pepper.

Instructions:

• Bake at 400 degrees Fahrenheit (200 degrees Celsius).

• Prepare a baking sheet with parchment paper and lay the salmon fillet on it.

• Marinate the salmon in a mixture of olive oil and lemon juice.

• Garlic powder, salt, and pepper should be used to season the fish.

• Mix olive oil, salt, and pepper with the vegetables in a separate bowl.

• Prepare a second baking sheet for the vegetables.

• In a preheated oven, bake the salmon and veggies for about 15-20 minutes, or until the salmon is flaky and the vegetables are soft.

• Roast the vegetables and serve them alongside the baked salmon for a healthy and delicious meal.

3. Stir-Fried Quinoa with Veggies:

• **Ingredients:**

• Toasted quinoa.

• Veggies galore (cauliflower, cabbage, cauliflower, carrots, onions, and more)

• Minced Garlic.

• Low-sodium tamari or soy sauce.

• Oil from sesame seeds.

• Green onions and sesame seeds can be added as a garnish.

Instructions:

• Sesame oil should be heated in a wok or big skillet over medium heat.

• Stir-fry the garlic mince for a minute to release its aroma.

• Put a variety of vegetables in a wok and stir-fry them until they are tender-crisp.

• Toss in some cooked quinoa and stir-fry everything together for a few minutes to blend the flavors.

• Stir-fry for one more minute after drizzling with low-sodium soy sauce or tamari.

• Turn off the heat and sprinkle on some sesame seeds and chopped green onion if you want.

• Prepare the quinoa and veggie stir-fry for a healthy and filling meal any time of day.

Make sure to modify the recipe to suit your tastes and dietary restrictions. You can adjust the flavor of these dishes by adding your favorite herbs, spices, or other ingredients. In addition, if your CLL treatment plan calls for any alterations to your diet, you should discuss these with your doctor or a trained dietitian.

Alternative Snacks

Some snack options that are safe for those with CLL are listed below.

1. Raw Produce:

• Eat some fruit, such as an apple, banana, orange, grape, or berry. They are a healthy source of sugar, fiber, and nutrients.

2. For the Greek Yogurt:

• Greek yogurt is a good source of protein and can be enhanced by adding fresh fruit or almonds for flavor and nutrition.

3. Crunchy Veggies with Creamy Hummus:

• Eat a handful of raw vegetables with a dollop of hummus as a snack. Examples include carrot sticks, cucumber slices, cherry tomatoes, and bell pepper strips. Fibre, vitamins, minerals, and good fats are all provided by this mix.

4. Protein-Rich Foods:

• Snack on some almonds, walnuts, pumpkin seeds, or sunflower seeds that have not been seasoned with salt. They provide a beneficial amount of protein, healthy fats, and essential vitamins and minerals.

5. Spreadable Nut Butter on Whole Grain Crackers:

• Use almond or peanut butter on a tablespoon of whole grain crackers for a healthy snack. This mixture has a delicious crunch, some beneficial fats, and some protein.

6. DIY Power Balls:

• Create your own energy balls with oats, nut butter, honey, and any other healthy ingredients you choose, such as chia seeds, flaxseeds, or dried fruits. These nutritious morsels can be eaten on the go.

7. Fresh Berries with Cottage Cheese:

• Have some fresh berries with your cottage cheese. Protein-rich cottage cheese and antioxidant-rich berries make for a delicious and filling snack.

8. Avocado and rice cakes:

• For a quick and healthy bite on the go, try spreading mashed avocado on whole grain rice cakes. Avocado provides heart-healthy fats and fiber, and rice cakes make a satisfying crunch.

9. Smoothies:

• Make a nutritious and delicious smoothie by blending together your favorite fruits and vegetables with some Greek yogurt and a beverage (such almond milk or coconut water). You have a lot of leeway in terms of component proportions to suit your individual palate.

Always think about how much you are eating and pay attention to when your body signals you are full. These nutritious snack options might help you feel full in between meals.

Modify the recipe to suit your tastes and dietary restrictions. Dietary restrictions and recommendations may be part of your CLL treatment plan; talk to your doctor or a certified dietitian for further information.

CHAPTER FIVE
Guidelines For Keeping Hydrated

Individuals managing CLL, like everyone else, can benefit from maintaining an appropriate water intake. To assist you maintain healthy levels of hydration, consider the following:

• Consume Adequate Fluids: Make sure you are getting enough water throughout the day. While eight cups (or 64 ounces) per day is the standard advice, everyone's water intake needs are different. To remind yourself to stay hydrated during the day, carry along a refillable water bottle.

• Pay Attention to Your Body's Cues If you are feeling thirsty, it is a good idea to quench your thirst by drinking some water. When you feel thirsty, your body is telling you that it needs water.

• Determine Your Level of Hydration by Observing Your Urine Color. Urine should be a light straw hue at most. Dehydration is indicated by darker urine, while overhydration is indicated by very light or clear urine.

• Distribute Your Fluid Intake Throughout the Day Rather than consuming a lot of fluid at once, spread it out throughout the day. That way, you will not have to worry about getting dehydrated or consuming too much water all at once.

• Foods That Keep You Hydrated: Eat plenty of water-rich foods like fruits and vegetables. Watermelon, cucumbers, oranges, strawberries, celery, and lettuce are all examples of fruits and vegetables. These foods also contain vital nutrients including vitamins and minerals, in addition to water.

• Caffeine and alcohol both have diuretic effects and should be consumed in moderation to prevent excessive fluid loss. Be sure to drink plenty of water to counteract the effects of caffeine and alcohol.

• Use alarms, phone applications, or any other form of reminder to ensure that you stay hydrated throughout the day. If you have a tendency to forget things or become distracted easily during the day, this may come in handy.

• Hydrate Before, During, and After Exercise If you engage in physical activity or exercise, it is important to stay hydrated by drinking water before, during, and after the activity.

Rehydrate by drinking water or a sports drink containing electrolytes to make up for fluid and electrolyte loss.

• Be aware of the temperature and humidity levels, and drink water or other fluids as needed. You may need to drink more fluids in hot weather or at high altitudes to make up for the loss of moisture from perspiration and the dry air.

• If you have any questions or concerns about your hydration habits, or if you have a medical condition that necessitates extra care, you should talk to your doctor.

Keep in mind that people have different water requirements depending on age, weight, degree of exercise, and health issues.

If you want advice on how much water to drink each day, it is best to talk to your doctor or a qualified dietitian about what is best for you.

Dietary Methods For Managing Adverse Effects Of Treatment

Dietary management of treatment-related side effects can be helpful for maximizing health and reducing distress. Common treatment side effects can be mitigated in a number of ways; however, it is always best to contact with your healthcare provider or a qualified dietitian for specific advice.

1. The Symptoms of Nausea and Vomiting:

• Eat several modest meals rather than three huge ones.

• Crackers, toast, rice, and boiling potatoes are all examples of bland, readily digestible items you should eat.

• If you are feeling nauseous, it is best to stay away from fatty, spicy, or highly-seasoned foods.

• Drink plenty of water or electrolyte-rich beverages (such ginger tea, peppermint tea, or sports drinks) to keep yourself hydrated.

• If you are feeling queasy, you might want to try ginger. It can be eaten in many different forms, including ginger tea, ginger candy, and cooked meals.

2. Sores in the mouth and trouble swallowing:

• Smoothies, soups, pureed veggies, and yogurt are all great options because they are soft and simple to swallow.

• If your mouth is sensitive, try to stay away from meals that are acidic, spicy, or have a rough texture.

• To alleviate mouth pain, try gargling with a saltwater solution before and after each meal.

• If you have trouble swallowing, try using a straw or a cup with a spout.

• Keep up with regular dental care by using a soft-bristled toothbrush and an alcohol-free mouthwash.

3. Altering Palate:

• To locate more appetizing foods, try varying the seasonings and preparation methods.

• Use citrus- or herb-based marinades to add depth of flavor to meats or veggies.

• To spice up your meals, experiment with various herbs and seasonings.

- It is possible that the milder flavors of cold or frozen foods make them more appealing to some people.

- Drink fluids regularly throughout the day, whether water or flavored drinks.

4. Fatigue:

- Eat a healthy, well-rounded diet that features a wide range of food groups.

- For long-lasting energy, whole grains, fruits, and vegetables should be eaten frequently.

- Chicken, fish, lentils, and tofu are all good examples of lean proteins that can help with both muscle maintenance and growth.

• Be sure to drink enough of water and other fluids every day.

• Reduce your coffee intake and replenish your energy with whole foods like fruits, nuts, and seeds.

5. Constipation or Diarrhea:

• For diarrhea, try the BRAT diet, which consists of bland meals like rice, applesauce, and toast.

• To keep your bowels regular, try eating more soluble fiber-rich foods like oats, boiled veggies, and well-cooked beans.

• If you have been experiencing diarrhea, it is important to replace the fluids you have lost by drinking lots of water.

• Foods high in fiber, such as whole grains, fruits, vegetables, and legumes, can help relieve constipation.

Maintain a regular exercise routine to promote regular bowel motions and other health benefits of physical activity.

It is important to communicate openly with your healthcare providers about any negative reactions you have had to treatment. They can tailor their advice and treatment to your specific needs. You can also benefit from the guidance of a certified dietician who specializes in oncology when it comes to managing treatment-related side effects and making the most of your nutritional intake.

CHAPTER SIX
Extra Lifestyle Factors To Think About

Chronic lymphocytic leukemia (CLL) management and general health support can be aided by various lifestyle factors beyond just nutrition. Extra suggestions for your way of life:

• Physical activity on a regular basis can help in many ways, from boosting energy and mood to keeping the weight down and increasing fitness levels. Before beginning an exercise regimen, you should talk to your doctor or healthcare provider to be sure it is safe for you to do so.

• Finding Effective Stress Management Strategies is Crucial to Your Physical and Emotional Health. Try some new methods of relieving stress, such yoga, deep breathing, mindfulness practices, or even just doing something you enjoy.

• Get enough sleep and stick to a regular sleep schedule as a top priority. Aim for 7 to 9 hours of quality sleep every night to aid in your health and speed up your recovery time.

• Seek out and keep in touch with loved ones and/or CLL-specific support groups who can listen to your struggles and help you feel less alone while you deal with CLL. It can be helpful to talk to other people who are going through the same things as you.

• Protect your skin from the sun and avoid getting too much sun to reduce your chances of getting skin cancer. Sunscreen with a high sun protection factor (SPF), protective clothing, and shade should all be used during the sun's peak hours.

• Do not smoke and drink alcohol in excess; both have bad effects on health and increase the likelihood of difficulties. Smokers should get help quitting, and alcoholics should drink only in moderation or as directed by their healthcare providers.

• Keep up with your regular appointments with your doctor for checkups, blood work, and imaging scans as directed. Your CLL's progression and response to therapy can be tracked with these checkups.

• Consistently taking prescribed medication as prescribed by your healthcare provider is an integral part of the treatment regimen. Talk to your doctor or healthcare provider about making changes or obtaining clarification if necessary.

• Keep an open line of contact with your healthcare team at all times. Quickly communicating any changes in your condition, worries, or treatment-related adverse effects can allow for the best possible care.

• Self-Care: Schedule time for activities that make you happy and calm down. Read, listen to music, practice hobbies, spend time in nature, or take a warm bath; these are all activities that have been shown to improve mental, emotional, and physical health.

Keep in mind that the experience of living with CLL is different for everyone. If you want tips and guidance tailored to your circumstances and treatment, talk to your healthcare providers. They can give you individualized advice to better manage your CLL.

Conclusion

Chronic lymphocytic leukemia (CLL) is a malignancy of the white blood cells that, as we have seen, necessitates intensive treatment. CLL management relies heavily on medical treatments and interventions, although leading a healthy lifestyle and eating well can help a great deal.

Focusing on nutrient-dense foods such as fruits, vegetables, whole grains, lean meats, and healthy fats is essential for a CLL-friendly diet. Vitamins, minerals, antioxidants, and fiber found in these foods have been shown to have positive effects on immunity, energy levels, and general well-being.

In addition, a healthy diet can help you deal with typical treatment-related side effects include nausea, mouth sores, altered taste sensations, drowsiness, and gastrointestinal difficulties.

You can reduce discomfort and increase nutrient intake by selecting the right foods, such as choosing bland, easily digestible foods or including particular cures like ginger for nausea.

Maintaining a healthy diet can be aided by eating a wide variety of

CLL-friendly foods and snacks, drinking plenty of water, and watching your serving amounts. Also, talk to your doctor or a certified dietitian for individualized recommendations based on your condition and treatment plan, as well as any dietary limitations you may have.

Lifestyle factors, such as exercise, stress reduction, rest, social support, and adherence to medical checkups, are also important in CLL management. You can improve your health, cope with treatment side effects, and increase your quality of life by following a holistic approach to CLL care that incorporates both medical and lifestyle factors.

Always consult with your medical staff to come up with a tailor-made treatment strategy. They will be able to guide you in the right direction, keep tabs on your progress, and change your treatment plan as needed to get you the greatest results.

THE END

Printed in Poland
by Amazon Fulfillment
Poland Sp. z o.o., Wrocław

36098665R00047